FAMILY ADDICTION

DEVELOP HEALTHY BOUNDARIES TO PROTECT YOUR HEALTH, FOSTER EMPATHY FOR THE ADDICT, AND HELP THEM FROM ROCK BOTTOM TO RECOVERY ROAD

JEREMY REYES

TABLE OF CONTENTS

INTRODUCTION

On a chilly evening in November, a family sat around their dining table – a scene that once symbolized warmth and unity now overshadowed by a palpable tension. At the head of the table sat Michael, whose journey into addiction had not only altered his life but had also sent ripples of change through his family. As tears welled in his mother's eyes and his father's hands clenched in anger and despair, Michael's sister, Sarah, reached across the table, her touch a silent plea for understanding and connection. This moment, fraught with pain, held an undercurrent of hope – a hope that things could change, that healing was possible, and that Michael could find his way back from the brink.

This book is born out of a deep desire to transform the narrative of helplessness that often surrounds families dealing with addiction into one of empowerment and action. It is for families like Michael's and for anyone who has felt the weight of a loved one's struggle with addiction. Through these pages, I aim to provide practical tools, strategies, and, most importantly, hope. By focusing on both the individual battling addiction and their family members, this book adopts a holistic approach, incorporating evidence-based strategies like Community Reinforcement and Family Training (CRAFT), Motivational Interviewing (MI), and Acceptance and Commitment Therapy (ACT). At its core, this book emphasizes empathy, understanding, and the significance of personal well-being.

Staggering statistics reveal that millions of families worldwide are navigating the complexities of addiction. In the United States alone, recent studies indicate that one in every three households is affected by some form of substance use disorder. This statistic underscores the urgency and relevance of our discussion, making it clear that the issue of family addiction is not isolated but widespread, touching the lives of many.

My connection to this topic is not just professional; it's personal. Having witnessed the impact of addiction within my own family, I understand the challenges and emotions that come with it. This experience has fueled my passion for supporting others through their journey, which grounds my approach to empathy and authenticity. As we explore this topic together, know that you are not alone. I stand with you as someone who has navigated these waters and as a guide.

In writing this book, I've committed to presenting approachable, compassionate, and hopeful information yet grounded in actionable advice. One of the key messages I hope to convey is the vital role of self-care for family members. Throughout the book, you'll find practical guidance on maintaining your health and well-being, ensuring you have the strength to support your loved one while also taking care of yourself.

The book is structured to guide you through understanding addiction, developing healthy boundaries, fostering empathy, and taking actionable steps toward recovery. While the journey through addiction and recovery is undoubtedly challenging, it is also filled with opportunities for growth, healing, and deeper connections.

I warmly invite you to join me on this journey. Though the road may be fraught with challenges, together, we can navigate the complexities of addiction with love, understanding, and practical strategies. By the end of this book, you will have a deeper understanding of addiction and be equipped with the tools needed to make a positive change in your and your loved ones' lives. Let's take this step forward together.

CHAPTER 1
UNTITLED

In the heart of every family touched by addiction lies a complex web of emotions, behaviors, and circumstances that defy simple explanations or solutions. The struggle with substance abuse, often seen merely as a series of poor choices or a lack of willpower, is deeply rooted in psychological underpinnings that stretch far beyond the individual's control or desire to change. From the shadows of trauma and stress to the subtle dynamics within a family, these factors collectively weave a narrative that is as unique as it is challenging. Understanding the psychological roots of addiction is akin to peeling an onion, layer by layer, each revealing its contribution to the whole picture. Within these layers, we uncover the "what" of addiction and the "why," offering insights that can lead to more empathetic approaches to healing and support.

1.1 The Psychological Roots of Addiction

Root Causes

The path leading to addiction often begins long before the first substance is ever consumed. Trauma, stress, and mental health disorders stand as towering gatekeepers on this road, shaping an individual's vulnerability to substance use. Traumatic experiences, particularly those endured during childhood, such as physical, emotional, or sexual abuse, can leave lasting scars that individuals struggle to heal. Stress, whether stemming from life changes, financial burdens, or interpersonal conflicts, further compounds this vulnerability, creating a fertile ground for addiction to take root. Mental health disorders, including depression, anxiety, and bipolar disorder, often exist in a precarious dance with substance use, each influencing and exacerbating the other. The National Institute on Drug Abuse highlights this interplay, noting that people with mood or anxiety disorders are twice as likely to suffer from drug addiction.

Emotional Pain

For many, substances offer a temporary haven from the relentless storm of emotional pain. This pain, often invisible to the outside world, becomes a constant companion that whispers promises of relief through the use of drugs or alcohol. The reality, though, is a far cry from the respite sought. Instead of healing, the cycle of addiction serves only to deepen the wounds, creating a feedback loop that is increasingly difficult to escape. The American Psychological Association underscores the role of emotional distress as a significant driver for substance use, pointing out that individuals often use drugs as a way to cope with complicated feelings or to self-medicate.

Behavioral Reinforcement

Once the cycle of use begins, the brain's reward system plays a pivotal role in reinforcing addictive behavior. This system, designed to recognize and encourage behaviors essential for survival, such as eating and socializing, becomes hijacked by substances that mimic or amplify the natural rewards of these activities. Dopamine, a neurotransmitter associated with pleasure and reward, floods the brain, creating a high that becomes intensely sought after. Over time, the brain's chemistry and structure adapt to this new normal, making the absence of the substance unpleasant and unbearable in many cases. The compulsion to use, driven by the brain's rewired reward system, transforms addiction from a choice to a necessity.

Family Dynamics

Nestled within the broader context of psychological factors are the intricate dynamics of family life, which can both mitigate and exacerbate the risk of addiction. On the one hand, a supportive, open, and communicative family environment can serve as a buffer against the pressures and pains that predispose individuals to substance use. On the other, patterns of enabling and codependency can unwittingly fuel the cycle of addiction. Enabling behaviors, characterized by actions that shield the individual from the consequences of their substance use, often stem from a desire to protect or help. However, these actions can decrease the individual's motivation for change. Codependency, where a family member's sense of purpose and self-worth becomes entangled with caring for the addicted individual, further complicates the family's ability to respond effectively. The Substance Abuse and Mental Health Services Administration (SAMHSA) emphasizes the importance of addressing these dynamics in treatment, highlighting how family therapy can play a crucial role in recovery by untangling these patterns and fostering healthier relationships.

In dissecting the psychological roots of addiction, it becomes clear that the journey toward substance use and the struggle with addiction is not merely a series of choices but a complex interplay of individual vulnerabilities, emotional pain, and environmental influences. This understanding is crucial, not just for the individuals and families navigating the depths of addiction but for society's approach to treatment and support. By shifting the focus from blame to empathy, from punishment to help, we can begin to unravel the threads of addiction and weave a new narrative of hope and healing.

1.2 How Addiction Rewires the Brain

The impact of addiction on the brain is profound and multifaceted, altering its very architecture and chemistry. This transformation not only fuels the cycle of addiction but also presents significant challenges for recovery. Understanding these changes is critical for both individuals struggling with addiction and their families, providing insights into the complexities of the condition and fostering a more compassionate approach to support and treatment.

Neurological Changes

Substance abuse initiates a cascade of changes within the brain, affecting both its structure and function. These substances interact with the brain's reward system, artificially elevating dopamine levels, a neurotransmitter associated with pleasure and motivation. Over time, the brain adjusts to these high dopamine levels by reducing its production and responsiveness, known as tolerance. This adaptation not only diminishes the individual's ability to experience pleasure from everyday activities but also compels them to use higher doses of the substance to achieve the same effect, further entrenching the cycle of addiction. Additionally, prolonged substance abuse can lead to alterations in areas of the brain responsible for judgment, decision-making, learning, and memory, complicating the recovery process by impairing the individual's ability to engage with treatment and make healthy choices.

Cravings and Compulsion

Distinguishing between physical dependency and psychological craving is pivotal in comprehending the full spectrum of addiction. Physical dependency refers to the body's adaptation to the presence of a substance, leading to withdrawal symptoms when use is reduced or stopped. These symptoms can range from discomfort to life-threatening, depending on the substance and duration of use. Psychological craving, however, stems from the brain's learned association between the substance and its effects, creating a powerful urge to use that can persist long after physical dependency has been addressed. This distinction underscores the dual nature of addiction as both a physiological and psychological condition, each aspect reinforcing the other and complicating the path to recovery.

Impact on Decision-Making

One of the most insidious effects of addiction is its impact on the brain's executive functions, including judgment, decision-making, impulse control, and emotional regulation. These functions, governed by the prefrontal cortex, are critical for planning, problem-solving, and self-control. Substance abuse can impair these abilities, making it increasingly difficult for individuals to weigh the long-term consequences of their actions against the immediate gratification of substance use. This impairment can lead to a cycle where poor decisions fuel further substance use, which in turn exacerbates the decline in executive function. This cycle hinders the individual's ability to seek and engage in treatment and affects their relationships, employment, and overall quality of life.

Reversibility

Despite the daunting challenges presented by these neurological changes, there is considerable hope for recovery and brain healing. Research has shown that the brain possesses a remarkable capacity for plasticity, allowing it to reorganize and form new connections in response to learning and experience. This plasticity means that, with sustained sobriety and engagement in recovery activities, individuals can begin to reverse some of the damage caused by addiction. Activities that promote brain health, such as exercise, healthy eating, mindfulness practices, and cognitive-behavioral therapies, can support this healing process. Additionally, engaging in new learning experiences and social connections can help to rebuild the brain's reward system, gradually restoring the ability to experience pleasure from everyday activities and reducing the reliance on substances for dopamine release.

The journey towards recovery is a testament to the human spirit's resilience and the brain's capacity to heal. As we navigate the complexities of addiction and its impact on the brain, it is imperative to approach those struggling with compassion, understanding, and support. By acknowledging the profound ways in which addiction rewrites the brain's functioning and structure, we can better appreciate the challenges faced by those in the grip of addiction and offer more effective interventions and encouragement. This understanding also serves as a beacon of hope, illuminating the path to recovery and the possibility of reclaiming a life unfettered by substance abuse.

1.3 The Family System and Addiction

Within the web of addiction's impact, the family system finds itself deeply entangled, each member assuming roles that, while protective in intent, often perpetuate the cycle of substance abuse. These roles emerge as silent responses to the chaos addiction brings, shaping interactions and expectations in ways that can both support and hinder recovery.

Roles within the Family

The dynamics within a family affected by addiction often lead to the adoption of specific roles by its members, each serving as a coping mechanism for the stresses and uncertainties brought about by substance abuse. These roles include:

- **The Enabler**, who, in their efforts to maintain peace and stability, may inadvertently shield the person with an addiction from the consequences of their actions. This role is usually filled by a partner or parent, driven by love yet caught in a cycle that prevents their loved one from facing the reality of their addiction.
- **The Hero**, usually an older child, strives for perfection in all areas of life as a counterbalance to the family's turmoil. Their achievements are a source of pride but also a mask for the pain and instability at home.
- **The Scapegoat** often acts out, drawing attention away from the family's core issue of addiction. Their rebellious behavior is a cry for help, yet it often reinforces the family's dysfunctional dynamics.
- **The Lost Child** withdraws, becoming quiet and reserved, to avoid adding to the family's burdens. Their silence, however, speaks volumes about the pain and neglect they experience.
- **The Mascot** uses humor as a deflection, lightening the family's mood and masking deep-seated fears and insecurities.

These roles, while offering temporary relief or distraction, can stifle genuine emotional expression and hinder the family's ability to confront and address the addiction head-on.

Communication Breakdown

Addiction weaves a complex web of secrecy and denial within the family, leading to a breakdown in healthy communication. Conversations that once flowed freely become fraught with tension, avoidance, and misunderstanding. Family members may tiptoe around the subject of addiction, fearing the conflict or emotional pain that addressing it might bring. This avoidance creates an environment where honest dialogue replaces silence or superficial exchanges, leaving each member feeling isolated and misunderstood. The lack of open communication prevents the family from coming together to support the person with an addiction in seeking help. It hinders their collective ability to heal and move forward.

Emotional Impact

The ripple effects of addiction on family members are profound, touching every aspect of their emotional well-being. The constant uncertainty, the cycle of hope followed by disappointment, and the shifts in family dynamics lead to a range of distressing emotions, including:

- Stress becomes a constant companion as family members navigate the unpredictability of addiction. This stress can manifest physically, leading to health issues that compound the family's challenges.
- Anxiety about the future, the well-being of the addicted loved one, and the stability of family life can be overwhelming, leading to sleepless nights and a pervasive sense of dread.

- Feelings of helplessness emerge as family members watch their loved one struggle with addiction, feeling powerless to effect change or halt the downward spiral.
- Guilt and blame often surface as family members question their actions or inactions, wondering if they could have done something differently to prevent the addiction or aid in recovery.

These emotions create a heavy burden that can strain relationships, disrupt daily life, and impede the family's functioning as a cohesive unit.

Path to Healing

Amidst the turmoil of addiction, family therapy emerges as a beacon of hope, offering a path to healing and recovery that encompasses the entire family system. This therapeutic approach recognizes the interconnectedness of family dynamics and addiction, aiming to:

- Unpack each family member's roles, exploring their origins and impact on the individual and the family. This understanding fosters a shift towards healthier interactions and roles that support recovery.
- Restore healthy communication, providing a safe space for expressing emotions, fears, and hopes. Through guided dialogue, family members learn to listen actively, speak honestly, and understand each other's perspectives, bridging the gaps that addiction has created.
- Address the emotional toll, helping each member to process their feelings, develop coping strategies, and

rebuild self-esteem. This emotional support is crucial for healing the wounds inflicted by addiction and strengthening the family's resilience.

- Realign the family system, shifting from dynamics that enable or exacerbate addiction to those that support sobriety and well-being. This realignment involves setting boundaries, establishing new patterns of interaction, and fostering a supportive environment conducive to recovery.

Family therapy, grounded in the principles of systemic healing, offers a comprehensive approach that not only aids the individual in overcoming addiction but also heals the family as a whole. Through this process, families can transform their pain and chaos into a foundation of strength, understanding, and hope, paving the way for a future free from the grip of addiction.

1.4 The Cycle of Denial in Families

Denial, a psychological defense mechanism, serves as a protective veil for families engulfed in the turmoil of addiction. It manifests as an inability or unwillingness to accept the reality of the situation, creating a barrier to acknowledging the problem and seeking help. Families often fall into this cycle, not out of a lack of love or concern, but as a means to cope with the overwhelming pain and fear that comes with admitting a loved one is struggling with addiction. This denial can take various forms, from minimizing the severity of the addiction to rationalizing the behavior or completely ignoring the signs.

Breaking free from the cycle of denial requires a delicate balance of understanding, patience, and action. Education plays a pivotal role in this process, shedding light on the nature of addiction as a complex disease rather than a moral failing. By learning about the biological, psychological, and social factors that contribute to addiction, families can begin to view the situation through a lens of compassion and understanding, reducing the stigma and shame that often fuels denial.

When done thoughtfully and with professional guidance, interventions can be a powerful tool in piercing the bubble of denial. They provide a structured opportunity for families to express their concerns and love while confronting the reality of addiction. The goal is not to place blame or provoke guilt but to open the door to acknowledgment and acceptance, laying the groundwork for recovery. However, interventions come with their challenges, including the potential for resistance or backlash from the person with addiction. Preparation, seeking advice from addiction professionals, timing, and setting can help mitigate these risks and increase the chances of a positive outcome.

Support systems are invaluable for families navigating the complex emotions and decisions that come with addressing addiction. Individual and family-based therapy offers a safe space for exploring feelings, healing relational wounds, and developing healthier communication and coping strategies. Support groups, such as Al-Anon or Nar-Anon, connect families with others who understand the unique struggles of loving someone with addiction, offering a sense of community, shared learning, and encouragement. These external resources not only aid in breaking the cycle of denial but also build resilience and hope for the future.

In moving past denial, families embark on a path of healing and recovery, not just for the individual with addiction but for themselves as well. This journey is marked by moments of challenge and growth, requiring a commitment to open-mindedness, learning, and support. By facing the reality of addiction together, families can navigate the road to recovery with strength, compassion, and a renewed sense of hope.

CHAPTER 2
SETTING HEALTHY BOUNDARIES

I magine a garden, your tranquility, growth, and beauty space. Now, think of boundaries as the fence around this garden. Without it, anything and anyone can trample through, leaving chaos in their wake. In the context of addiction, boundaries serve a similar purpose. They protect the emotional, physical, and financial well-being of both the individual and the family from the unpredictable turmoil addiction can create. This chapter addresses how to define, establish, and maintain these protective fences, ensuring the garden — your family — thrives even in adversity.

2.1 Concept of Boundaries

Boundaries are the rules and limits we set for ourselves within relationships. They are crucial in any family dynamic but become even more so when dealing with addiction. Think of boundaries not as barriers to keep loved ones out but as clear lines safeguarding both parties' well-being. Without them, the chaos of addiction can quickly upend the family balance, leading to resentment, burnout, and a host of other issues.

Types of Boundaries

Boundaries come in many forms, each serving a unique purpose:

- **Emotional Boundaries** protect your mental health by limiting exposure to emotionally harmful behaviors, such as verbal abuse or manipulation.
- **Physical Boundaries** involve personal space and physical contact, ensuring safety and comfort.
- **Financial Boundaries** prevent the financial strain of addiction from consuming the family's resources, setting clear limits on money management and support.

Understanding these types helps craft a comprehensive boundary plan that addresses all aspects of family well-being.

Establishing Boundaries

Setting boundaries is a step-by-step process:

1. **Identify Needs:** Start by pinpointing your need to feel safe, respected, and healthy. Is it more personal space? Limits on financial support? Understanding your needs is the foundation of effective boundaries.
2. **Communicate Clearly:** Once you know your needs, express them to your loved one. Use "I" statements to frame these needs from your perspective, avoiding blame.

3. **Be Consistent:** Consistency is vital. Boundaries only work if they are upheld consistently. This means not making exceptions or bending the rules, as doing so can send mixed messages.
4. **Prepare for Pushback:** It's natural to meet resistance. Stay firm and reiterate your boundaries calmly and clearly.
5. **Adjust as Needed:** As situations change, be willing to revisit and adjust your boundaries. This flexibility allows the boundary framework to grow with your family's evolving needs.

Challenges to Boundaries

While setting boundaries is crucial, it's not without its challenges:

- **Guilt:** Many families feel guilt when setting boundaries, feeling they are abandoning their loved ones. It's important to remember that boundaries are a form of care ensuring the health of all parties involved.
- **Manipulation:** An addicted loved one might try to manipulate boundaries to suit their desires. Recognizing manipulation tactics and standing firm in your decisions helps mitigate this challenge.
- **Internal Family Resistance:** Not all family members may agree on the boundaries set, leading to internal conflict. Open, honest discussions about the importance and purpose of these boundaries help align everyone's perspectives.

Setting boundaries in the context of addiction is akin to planting a garden. It requires patience, care, and constant nurturing. With clear, consistent boundaries, families can create a space where healing is possible, allowing everyone to grow and thrive despite the challenges addiction may bring.

2.2 Practical Steps to Establish Boundaries

Navigating the landscape of family addiction requires a map to avoid the pitfalls that can disrupt the balance and harmony at home. Establishing boundaries is akin to drawing this map, marking safe passages, and noting areas to avoid. This section outlines steps that families can follow to create a practical, actionable boundary plan that respects the needs and limits of all family members.

Identifying Needs

The initial step in setting boundaries involves profoundly reflecting on what each family member requires to feel secure, respected, and emotionally healthy. It's a time for honest introspection, where you ask yourself what behaviors you can accept and what actions cross the line. For some, this might mean no substance use in the house, while for others, it could involve limitations on financial assistance or specific expectations around behavior and communication.

To facilitate this process, consider:

- Creating a list of non-negotiables is critical for maintaining a healthy family environment.
- Discussing these needs as a family, where each member can voice their requirements and concerns.

- Remembering that needs can differ significantly between family members and finding common ground is vital.

Communication Techniques

Once needs are identified, effectively conveying them becomes paramount. Communication should always be rooted in empathy and understanding, recognizing that the addicted family member is facing their own set of challenges. However, being assertive is also crucial, ensuring your message is clear and direct.

Strategies for effective communication include:

- Planning what you want to say ahead of time, focusing on clarity, and the avoidance of ambiguity.
- Choosing a calm, neutral time and setting to discuss boundaries, away from the heat of conflict or high emotion.
- Employing active listening, showing your loved one that you value their perspective and are open to dialogue.
- Using "I" statements to express how specific behaviors affect you personally reduces the likelihood of defensiveness or hostility in response.

Enforcement Strategies

With boundaries communicated, the focus shifts to enforcement — a challenging yet vital component of the boundary-setting process. Consistent enforcement underscores the seriousness of the boundaries and helps establish a framework of predictability and trust within the family.

Consider the following when enforcing boundaries:

- Preparing for initial resistance and having a plan in place for how to respond calmly and firmly.
- Implementing natural consequences for boundary violations directly related to the breach will help underscore the importance of respecting family rules.
- Engaging in regular family check-ins to discuss how well the boundaries are working and address any issues or feelings that arise.
- Seeking external support, such as from a therapist or support group, to provide guidance and reinforcement during challenging moments.

Adjusting Boundaries

The dynamic nature of addiction means that the family's needs and circumstances can change over time, necessitating adjustments to previously set boundaries. Flexibility allows the family to adapt to these changes, ensuring that boundaries remain relevant and supportive of everyone's well-being.

To adjust boundaries effectively:

- Monitor the impact of current boundaries on family dynamics and individual well-being, noting any areas of tension or difficulty.
- Hold family meetings to discuss these observations and consider whether adjustments are needed to support recovery and family health better.

- Be open to feedback from all family members, including the person with addiction, acknowledging that their recovery journey may also shift their needs and capabilities.
- Ensure that all communicate and understand any changes, maintaining the clarity and consistency essential for effective boundary management.

Through these steps, families can develop a robust framework of boundaries that protect and nurture all involved, adapting as needed to the ever-changing landscape of addiction and recovery. This process, though challenging, fosters an environment of respect, safety, and mutual support, laying the groundwork for healing and positive change.

2.3 Communicating Your Boundaries Effectively

Navigating the complex waters of addiction within the family necessitates clear communication, especially when it comes to expressing boundaries. This facet of interaction isn't merely about stating rules; it's an art that intertwines respect, clarity, and empathy. How boundaries are communicated can significantly influence their reception and adherence, making the difference between a step forward in healing and an unnecessary rift in the family fabric.

Language Matters

The words we choose and how we frame our messages are pivotal in how our boundaries are perceived and respected. Utilizing "I" statements becomes a powerful tool in this regard. By focusing on your feelings and experiences rather than attributing blame, you facilitate a conversation that's less likely to escalate into defensiveness or conflict. For instance, saying, "I feel overwhelmed when I have to cover your expenses due to your addiction," centers the conversation on your feelings and needs, inviting understanding rather than inciting guilt or defensiveness.

Moreover, the clarity of your message ensures there's no room for misunderstanding. Ambiguity can lead to assumptions and expectations that misalign with your intentions. Therefore, articulate your boundaries with as much precision as possible, leaving no doubt about what you expect and why it's important to you.

Timing and Setting

The impact of your words also hinges on when and where you choose to express them. Discussing boundaries during a crisis or an emotionally charged moment can lead to heightened tensions and ineffective communication. Opt for a calm, neutral moment when you and your loved one are more likely to engage in a productive dialogue. The setting also plays a role; a private, comfortable space where you won't be interrupted or distracted allows for a level of intimacy and focus that is conducive to understanding and acceptance.

Expecting Resistance

Anticipating resistance is a realistic and necessary part of setting boundaries with a loved one struggling with addiction. The discomfort and pushback you might receive are not always reflections of disregard for your needs but can manifest the struggle your loved one is facing. When met with resistance, maintain your composure and reassert your boundaries with empathy. It's helpful to recognize the difference between a genuine need for clarification and attempts to negotiate your boundaries away. Stand firm, yet remain open to discussing how these boundaries serve the well-being of everyone involved.

At times, resistance can escalate to more intense reactions. In these instances, it's crucial to safeguard your emotional well-being. Remind yourself that setting boundaries is not only for your health but also for the ultimate benefit of your loved one. It's about creating an environment where recovery can flourish.

Seeking Support

The journey of setting and maintaining boundaries can be walked with others. Seeking support from external sources can bolster your resolve and provide you with additional strategies for effective communication. Family therapy offers a structured environment where a professional can guide the conversation, ensuring that boundaries are communicated in a way that's constructive and understood by all parties. The therapist can also mediate any resistance or conflict that arises, helping to navigate through the emotions and reactions of these discussions.

Support groups present another avenue for reinforcement. Sharing experiences with others facing similar challenges can offer new perspectives and insights into effective communication strategies. It's a space where you can find understanding, encouragement, and validation from individuals who genuinely grasp the nuance of your situation. These groups can also remind you that you're not alone, providing a sense of community and shared resilience.

Moreover, literature and online resources focused on addiction recovery and family dynamics can equip you with knowledge and techniques to enhance your communication skills. Educating yourself on the nature of addiction and the psychological aspects of boundary setting can deepen your understanding of what effective communication in this context entails.

In sum, communicating boundaries within the milieu of addiction is a delicate balance of clarity, empathy, and timing, supported by a foundation of self-care and external support. It's a process that fosters an environment conducive to healing, growth, and, ultimately, recovery.

2.4 Boundaries and Self-Care: Balancing Acts

Navigating the complex dynamics of addiction within a family often means putting the needs of a loved one first. However, amid this challenging landscape, it's critical to recognize the importance of your well-being. Recognizing that self-care is not selfish but rather a necessary aspect of supporting others is the first step towards creating a balanced life. Here, we'll explore how setting boundaries is an act of self-care, ways to manage feelings of guilt, and strategies to balance supporting your loved one with preserving your well-being.

Self-Care as a Priority

When you're preoccupied with the well-being of a family member struggling with addiction, your own needs can quickly fall by the wayside. However, neglecting self-care can lead to burnout, resentment, and a decrease in your ability to provide support. Viewing boundary-setting as an act of self-care is essential. It allows you to protect your energy and emotional health, ensuring you're in a better position to offer support. Remember, you cannot pour from an empty cup. Prioritizing self-care enables you to replenish your resources so you're more effective in helping your loved one.

Guilt and Self-Compassion

It's common to experience guilt when setting boundaries as if you're somehow letting your loved one down. This guilt can be overwhelming, but it's essential to recognize it as a natural response to a difficult situation. Cultivating self-compassion involves acknowledging these feelings without judgment and reminding yourself of the necessity and validity of your boundaries. Strategies to foster self-compassion include:

- **Mindfulness practices:** Engaging in mindfulness can help you recognize and accept your feelings of guilt without being overwhelmed by them.
- **Positive self-talk:** Replace critical or guilt-laden thoughts with kinder, more supportive messages.
- **Seeking support:** Talking with others who understand your situation can provide perspective and validation, reducing feelings of guilt.

Balancing Support and Self-Preservation

Finding an equilibrium between supporting your loved one and maintaining your health and happiness is crucial. This balance does not imply caring less; instead, it means not allowing your well-being to be consumed by your loved one's addiction. Establishing and maintaining boundaries is vital to this balance. It's also important to recognize that you have limits and that it's okay to say no or to ask for help when needed. Balancing support with self-preservation means:

- Knowing your limits and communicating them.
- Recognizing signs of physical and emotional exhaustion and taking steps to address them.
- Allowing yourself to take breaks and stepping back when necessary to recharge.

Examples of Self-Care Practices

Incorporating self-care practices into your daily routine can significantly impact your ability to cope with the challenges of a loved one's addiction. Examples of self-care practices include:

- **Physical activity:** Regular exercise, whether a daily walk, yoga, or a more intense workout, can reduce stress and improve mood.
- **Hobbies and interests:** Engaging in activities you enjoy can provide a much-needed distraction and a sense of normalcy.
- **Healthy routines:** Establishing routines around sleep, nutrition, and relaxation can bolster your physical and mental health.
- **Social connections:** Spending time with friends and engaging in social activities can offer support and reduce feelings of isolation.
- **Professional support:** Seeking therapy or counseling can provide a space to process emotions and develop coping strategies.

In conclusion, setting boundaries is not just about creating limits for your loved one; it's an act of self-care that preserves your well-being. By prioritizing self-care, managing guilt with compassion, and finding a balance between supporting your loved one and caring for yourself, you create a healthier environment for everyone involved. As we move forward, remember the importance of these practices not only for your health but also as a foundation for the ongoing support and care you offer to your loved one struggling with addiction.

CHAPTER 3
FOSTERING A FOUNDATION
FOR RECOVERY

Imagine a house where every room is filled with different tunes playing simultaneously. In one room, classical music underscores a serene atmosphere, while just a wall away, heavy metal shakes the very foundations of the house. This cacophony mirrors a family navigating addiction without a unified understanding or approach. It's within this chaos that the necessity for a supportive family environment becomes clear. It's not about silencing any tune but finding harmony where each note contributes to a more beautiful symphony.

Creating this harmonious environment involves open dialogue, education, empowerment through knowledge, and the strategic use of family therapy. These elements act as instruments in orchestrating a setting conducive to recovery and long-term well-being for both the individual struggling with addiction and their family.

3.1 Promoting Open Dialogue

Open, honest communication is the cornerstone of a supportive family environment. It's about creating a space where family can share fears, hopes, frustrations, and victories without judgment. To foster this:

- **Set regular family meetings:** Pick a consistent time each week for check-ins, establishing a routine everyone can rely on.
- **Use active listening:** Show that you value the speaker's perspective by summarizing their points and asking follow-up questions.
- **Encourage all to participate:** Sometimes, the quietest are the most affected, and gentle encouragement can help them open up.

This dialogue nurtures trust and understanding, making it easier to navigate the ups and downs of recovery together.

Educating the Family

Misconceptions about addiction abound, often leading to stigma and misunderstanding. Education dispels these myths, paving the way for empathy and informed support. Consider the following steps:

- **Utilize reputable sources:** Websites, books, and pamphlets from trusted organizations provide accurate information about addiction.
- **Attend workshops and seminars:** Many community centers and hospitals offer sessions on understanding addiction and how to support recovery.

- **Learn together:** Make it a family activity to read an article or watch a documentary about addiction, followed by a discussion.

Armed with knowledge, the family can stand unified in their approach to supporting their loved one, reducing the sense of isolation that addiction often brings.

Empowering through Knowledge

Beyond understanding addiction itself, knowing how to support a loved one's recovery journey actively is crucial. This empowerment comes from accessing a variety of resources:

- **Recommendations for books:** Create a family book club with titles focused on addiction recovery and resilience.
- **Workshops and seminars:** Look for events that provide strategies for supporting loved ones through recovery.
- **Online courses:** Many platforms offer free or low-cost classes on topics ranging from communication strategies to understanding the science of addiction.

Equipped with strategies and insights, families can navigate the recovery process more effectively, becoming proactive participants rather than feeling sidelined.

Role of Family Therapy

Family therapy offers a structured approach to addressing not just the addiction but the underlying issues within the family dynamic that may contribute to or exacerbate the situation. This therapy:

- **Improves communication:** A therapist can help family members learn how to communicate their needs and feelings more effectively.
- **Addresses underlying issues:** Therapy sessions can uncover and work through problems contributing to stress within the family.
- **Strengthens the family unit:** By working through these issues together, families can emerge stronger and more united in their approach to recovery.

Engaging in family therapy demonstrates a commitment to healing not just the individual but the family as a whole.

In implementing these strategies, families transform from a collection of individuals struggling with the chaos of addiction into a united front. This shift doesn't erase the challenges of addiction, but it equips families with the tools to face them together, fostering an environment where recovery can truly flourish.

3.2 The Role of Self-Care for Caregivers

Caring for a loved one with an addiction can often lead to a path where the caregiver's well-being is inadvertently placed on the back burner. The focus shifts so intently on the person in need that signs of personal strain may go unnoticed until they become severe. Recognizing these signs early, setting personal limits, adopting self-care practices, and embracing external support networks are not just acts of self-preservation but are crucial for sustaining the ability to provide care.

Identifying Signs of Caregiver Burnout

The initial step in averting caregiver burnout involves recognizing its early warning signs. These can manifest as physical symptoms like chronic fatigue, changes in appetite, or sleep disturbances. Emotionally, caregivers may experience heightened anxiety, depression, or irritability. A sense of feeling overwhelmed or decreased satisfaction from activities that once brought joy can also signify the onset of burnout. Acknowledging these symptoms as legitimate and addressing them can prevent the spiral into deeper emotional and physical exhaustion.

Establishing Personal Boundaries

For caregivers, setting personal boundaries is not a negotiable aspect of their role; it's necessary. These boundaries help define what they can provide, safeguarding their mental and physical health. Effective boundary-setting involves:

- Understanding your limits by reflecting on what aspects of caregiving contribute to feelings of stress or resentment.
- Communicating these boundaries clearly to the addiction family members, ensuring they understand the necessity behind these limits.
- Enforcing boundaries means saying no or stepping back consistently when certain lines are approached or crossed.

These steps help caregivers maintain a sense of self amidst the demands of caregiving, preventing resentment and burnout.

Self-Care Strategies

Incorporating self-care strategies into daily routines can significantly bolster a caregiver's resilience. These strategies vary widely, allowing for personalization based on individual preferences and lifestyles. Key strategies include:

- Mindfulness practices like meditation or deep-breathing exercises can reduce stress and enhance emotional regulation.
- Physical activity, whether a brisk walk, yoga, or an exercise class, is necessary to improve overall health and reduce stress.
- Engaging in hobbies that bring joy and provide an escape from caregiving responsibilities, such as painting, gardening, or reading.
- Maintaining social connections by spending time with friends and family who provide emotional support and a sense of normalcy outside the caregiving role.

Implementing these practices helps caregivers recharge, offering a buffer against the stress associated with their role.

Seeking Support

Recognizing when to seek external support is a testament to a caregiver's strength, not a sign of weakness. Various forms of support are available:

- Counseling or therapy can provide a space to process emotions, cope with stress, and strategize on managing caregiving responsibilities.

- Support groups offer a community of individuals facing similar challenges, providing empathy, understanding, and practical advice.
- Community resources, such as respite care services, can offer temporary relief, allowing caregivers to take necessary breaks.

Utilizing these resources can provide caregivers with the support needed to sustain their well-being and their ability to care for their loved ones effectively.

Caregivers can create a sustainable balance by recognizing the early signs of burnout, establishing and maintaining personal boundaries, adopting tailored self-care practices, and leveraging external support networks. This balance ensures they remain healthy and resilient, capable of providing the compassionate care their loved one needs while not losing sight of their well-being.

3.3 Leveraging Community Resources

In the landscape of addiction recovery, the phrase "it takes a village" couldn't be more apt. While the family unit forms the core support system, extending this network to include community resources, friends, extended family, and professionals significantly enriches the support available. This broader network not only brings diverse perspectives and resources but also helps dilute the intensity of managing addiction within the confined space of the immediate family.

Navigating Support Services

The first step towards leveraging community resources is identifying what's out there. Local support groups, addiction services, and educational programs offer a wealth of knowledge and assistance. For many, the challenge lies not in the absence of these resources but in pinpointing which ones align with their needs. Here's how to navigate this landscape:

- **Research local organizations:** Many communities have organizations dedicated to addiction recovery. These communities are found through internet searches, local health clinics, or community centers.
- **Ask for recommendations:** Healthcare providers, therapists, and social workers can provide valuable suggestions on reputable local services.
- **Attend community events:** Often, local events related to health and wellness can connect you to organizations that offer support for families dealing with addiction.

The goal is to compile a list of resources that feel like a good fit for your family's specific situation.

Building a Support Network

The strength of a support network lies in its diversity. Friends, extended family, and professionals each bring unique insights and forms of support. Building this network involves:

- **Openly communicating needs:** Sharing with friends and extended family what you're going through opens the door for them to offer support.
- **Joining support groups:** Whether a local Al-Anon or a similar support group, connecting with others in similar situations can provide solace and practical advice.
- **Reaching out to professionals:** Addiction counselors, therapists, and social workers can offer guidance, not just for the person struggling with addiction but for the family as a whole.

This network becomes a safety net, offering emotional support, practical advice, and a sense of community that can be invaluable during challenging times.

Online Resources and Social Media

The digital age brings access to a global support community. Online forums, social media groups, and reputable websites offer a wealth of information and connections accessed from the comfort of your home. Here's how to make the most of these resources:

- **Identify reputable websites:** Look for sites affiliated with recognhgized health organizations or those that offer evidence-based information.
- **Join online forums and groups:** Platforms like Facebook and Reddit host numerous groups for families affected by addiction. These can be a source of support, advice, and camaraderie.
- **Follow addiction recovery blogs:** Many blogs offer insights into the journey of recovery from both the

perspective of those battling addiction and their families. These can offer comfort, inspiration, and practical advice.

Online resources break down geographical barriers, allowing families to find support and information that might not be available locally.

Collaboration with Professionals

Working closely with addiction professionals, therapists, and counselors ensures a cohesive approach to supporting your loved one's recovery. Collaboration can take many forms, from seeking input on the best local resources to involving professionals in family meetings for guidance. Here's how to effectively collaborate:

- **Maintain open lines of communication:** Keeping therapists and counselors informed of the family's challenges and progress ensures they can offer tailored advice and support.
- **Ask for resources:** Professionals can recommend books, workshops, and support groups to aid the family's understanding and coping strategies.
- **Consider family therapy:** Involving a therapist in regular family sessions can help address underlying issues, improve communication, and strengthen the family unit as a support system.

This collaboration not only enriches the family's toolkit for managing addiction but also ensures a unified front in supporting the loved one on their path to recovery.

Families can create a comprehensive support system by weaving together these various strands of support—community resources, a broader support network, online avenues, and professional collaboration. This system not only aids in navigating the complexities of addiction but also promotes a healthier balance within the family, ensuring that each member, not just the individual struggling with addiction, receives the support they need.

3.4 Navigating the Recovery System: A Primer for Families

The path to recovery is as varied as the individuals walking it, with no one-size-fits-all solution. Families often find themselves at a crossroads, trying to decide which recovery option will best suit their loved one's needs. It's a decision that carries weight, as the right choice can significantly influence the success of the recovery process.

Understanding Different Recovery Pathways

The landscape of recovery options is vast, ranging from intensive inpatient programs to flexible outpatient services and supportive self-help groups. Each recovery option has its strengths and is designed to meet different needs at various stages of recovery.

- Inpatient treatment offers a structured environment, providing round-the-clock care and support. This option is particularly beneficial for those who need a break from their daily environment to focus entirely on recovery.

- Outpatient programs allow individuals to continue their daily lives while receiving treatment. Programs can include therapy sessions, support groups, and educational workshops.
- Self-help groups, such as Alcoholics Anonymous or Narcotics Anonymous, foster a community of support among individuals who share similar experiences. These groups provide a platform for sharing strategies and encouragement.

Deciding on the best path involves considering the severity of the addiction, the individual's circumstances, and their readiness for change. Open discussions within the family and consultations with addiction professionals can guide this decision-making process.

The Role of Detoxification

Detoxification marks the first step toward recovery, clearing the body of substances. It's a critical phase that can be physically challenging and requires medical supervision to manage withdrawal symptoms safely.

During detox, families should prepare for:

- **Withdrawal symptoms:** These can range from mild discomfort to severe physical reactions. Understanding these symptoms can help families provide support and encouragement.
- **Emotional fluctuations:** Alongside physical symptoms, individuals may experience intense emotions. Patience and empathy from family

members can make a significant difference during
this volatile time.

- **The need for professional supervision:** Detox should
never be attempted alone. Medical professionals can
ensure the process is as safe and comfortable as
possible.

Insurance and Financial Considerations

The financial aspect of recovery treatment concerns many
families. Navigating insurance coverage and understanding
the available options can alleviate some of the stress associated with these costs.

- **Review your insurance policy:** Start by
understanding what your policy covers regarding
addiction treatment; this might include inpatient care,
outpatient therapy, and medication.
- **Explore payment plans and scholarships:** Many
treatment centers offer payment plans or scholarships
to help cover costs. Don't hesitate to ask about these
options.
- **Seek advice from professionals:** Financial counselors
or case managers within treatment centers can guide
you in managing the costs associated with recovery.

While financial considerations are important, they should not
deter families from seeking treatment. Resources are available
to help manage these expenses, ensuring recovery remains
accessible.

Long-term Recovery Planning

Recovery extends far beyond the initial treatment phase, requiring ongoing support and vigilance to maintain sobriety. Planning for long-term recovery involves:

- **Relapse prevention strategies:** Identifying triggers and developing coping strategies can help prevent relapse. Strategies might include regular therapy sessions, continued support group participation, and healthy activities.
- **Building a supportive environment:** A stable home environment is crucial in long-term recovery. This environment includes open communication, continued education about addiction, and encouragement for healthy habits.
- **Ongoing support:** The need for support doesn't end once formal treatment concludes. Continued involvement in self-help groups or therapy can provide the reinforcement needed to maintain sobriety.

Recovery is a continuous process that evolves. By planning for the long term, families can create a framework that supports sustained sobriety, offering their loved ones the best chance for a fulfilling life post-addiction.

As we close this chapter, it's clear that navigating the recovery system requires patience, research, and a willingness to adapt. From understanding the diverse treatment options and the critical role of detoxification to managing financial considerations and planning for long-term recovery, each step is a building block towards a healthier future. The journey of recovery is a testament to the resilience of both the individual and their family, underscored by love, support, and the shared goal of a life free from addiction. As we move forward, the focus shifts to sustaining recovery and the family's ongoing role in this enduring process.

CHAPTER 4
TRANSFORMING STRATEGIES INTO FAMILY STRENGTHS

In the maze of addiction recovery, feeling lost is more common than finding one's way on the first attempt. It's like navigating through a dense forest without a compass, where every turn looks promising yet leads back to square one. However, when families arm themselves with a map of evidence-based strategies—CRAFT, MI, and ACT—they suddenly find themselves holding a compass, a guide through uncharted territories. This chapter highlights these approaches not as abstract theories but as practical tools for everyday life, transforming them from strategies into natural strengths within the family unit.

4.1 Overview of Each Approach

Community Reinforcement and Family Training (CRAFT), Motivational Interviewing (MI), and Acceptance and Commitment Therapy (ACT) stand as three pillars supporting the bridge to recovery.

- **CRAFT** focuses on positive reinforcement, encouraging behaviors that lead to sobriety. It's about understanding what motivates change and using these insights to guide a loved one toward recovery.
- **MI** hinges on the art of conversation, using empathy and strategic questioning to inspire the motivation to change. It's about listening and responding in ways that make a loved one consider their choices and the possibility of a different path.
- **ACT** dives into accepting what cannot be changed, committing to what can be, and taking action based on personal values. It's about embracing the present moment, understanding personal values, and moving forward purposefully.

Each approach brings its unique strengths to the table, yet they all share a common goal: to support families and individuals in navigating the journey of addiction recovery.

Applicability to Family Situations

It's one thing to understand these approaches in theory; it's another to see how they fit into the jigsaw puzzle of daily family life.

- **CRAFT** comes into play when considering how to respond to a loved one's behaviors. For instance, recognizing and celebrating small victories, like attending a therapy session, reinforces positive steps toward recovery.
- **MI** proves invaluable in conversations that could quickly turn confrontational. By asking open-ended questions and reflecting on a loved one's responses,

families can foster a dialogue that encourages self-reflection and consideration of change.

- **ACT** becomes a guiding principle in managing the emotional rollercoaster of addiction. It helps families focus on their values, like love and support, guiding their actions and responses to their loved ones.

Integrating these strategies into family life means moving beyond the textbook, applying them in situations as varied as discussing treatment options, setting boundaries, or simply sharing a quiet moment of connection.

Integrating Strategies into Daily Life

Integrating CRAFT, MI, and ACT into daily interactions doesn't require a drastic overhaul of how families communicate or support each other. It's about tweaking the approaches and making minor adjustments that can significantly impact them.

- For **CRAFT** might be as simple as changing how you greet your loved one when they come home, focusing on positive engagement rather than diving into problem-solving mode.
- With **MI** could involve shifting from why questions, which can imply judgment, to how questions, which invite exploration and understanding.
- **ACT** integration might mean starting family meetings with a brief mindfulness exercise and setting a tone of presence and openness for the following discussions.

These small steps can lead to a profound shift in the family dynamic, creating an environment where recovery is supported and every family member feels heard and valued.

Evidence of Effectiveness

The proof, as they say, is in the pudding. Research and case studies highlight the effectiveness of CRAFT, MI, and ACT in the realm of addiction recovery. For example, a study published in the Journal of Substance Abuse Treatment found that families using CRAFT strategies were more successful in engaging their loved ones in treatment compared to those using traditional interventions. Similarly, MI has been shown to enhance motivation for change, leading to better outcomes in substance abuse treatment. ACT's emphasis on acceptance and commitment has been linked to improved mental health and resilience, both crucial for families navigating the challenges of addiction.

These findings offer families not just hope but a roadmap. They underscore the potential of these strategies to make a tangible difference in the recovery process, providing the individual and their family with the tools to build a stronger, healthier future together.

As families begin to weave CRAFT, MI, and ACT into the fabric of their daily lives, they transform theoretical strategies into practical strengths. This chapter aims to demystify these approaches, presenting them not as clinical interventions but as accessible, adaptable tools for families. In doing so, it offers a beacon of light, guiding families through the complexities of addiction recovery and toward a path of healing and hope.

4.2 Practical Exercises Based on CRAFT

The heart of the Community Reinforcement and Family Training (CRAFT) approach lies in its practical application, offering families a set of tools tailored to encourage positive change. These exercises have been designed to support the individual in recovery and strengthen the family unit, promoting a nurturing and supportive environment.

Identifying Positive Reinforcements

Positive reinforcements are crucial in motivating behavior change. Identifying these involves understanding what motivates your loved one and using these insights to encourage steps toward sobriety.

- Start by listing activities or rewards that your loved one enjoys. These could range from simple pleasures like a favorite meal to more significant rewards like attending a sports event together.
- Next, connect these rewards to specific positive behaviors you want to encourage, such as attending a counseling session or participating in family activities.
- Implement a plan where these rewards are consistently given in response to positive behaviors. The rewards must be immediate and directly linked to the behavior to reinforce the connection between action and positive outcomes.

Developing Communication Skills

Effective communication is the cornerstone of the CRAFT approach, fostering an atmosphere where open dialogue can flourish. Enhancing these skills involves exercises that focus on active listening, expressing concern without judgment, and clear articulation of thoughts and feelings.

- Practice active listening by having family members share something about their day, with others focusing solely on listening, then accurately summarizing what was said. This exercise helps improve empathy and understanding.
- Role-play scenarios where you express concerns about your loved one's behavior. Focus on using "I feel" statements rather than accusations to communicate how their actions impact you emotionally.
- Engage in daily check-ins with each family member, dedicating a few minutes to share feelings, concerns, or simply how the day went. This routine fosters a habit of open communication.

Problem-Solving Techniques

Facing challenges together and finding solutions as a unit is another aspect CRAFT emphasizes. These techniques aim to involve the addicted individual in problem-solving, strengthening their sense of agency and responsibility.

- Introduce a weekly family problem-solving meeting. Present a challenge the family faces (unrelated to addiction) and brainstorm solutions together. This meeting fosters a collaborative atmosphere and enhances problem-solving skills.

- For challenges directly related to addiction, use a structured approach to explore solutions. First, define the problem clearly. Then, brainstorm potential solutions without judgment. Finally, evaluate the pros and cons of each solution before deciding on the best course of action together.
- Keep a family problem-solving journal. Document the challenges faced, the solutions tried, and the outcomes. This journal helps track progress and understand what strategies work best for your family.

Self-Care Activities for Families

CRAFT emphasizes the importance of self-care for families, recognizing that supporting a loved one through addiction can be a taxing experience. Incorporating self-care into the family routine ensures that everyone's well-being is maintained.

- Schedule regular family self-care days where each member chooses an activity that promotes relaxation and enjoyment. This day could be anything from a movie night to a day out in nature.
- Start a family gratitude journal. Each day, have every family member write down one thing they are grateful for. This practice encourages a focus on the positive aspects of life, enhancing overall well-being.
- Engage in regular physical activities like walks, bike rides, or yoga sessions. Physical well-being is closely linked to mental health; doing these activities together strengthens family bonds.

- Organize family workshops or sessions on stress management techniques. Learning and practicing these techniques can provide everyone with the tools to manage stress more effectively.

Through these exercises, families can harness the principles of CRAFT, transforming them into tangible actions that support recovery and strengthen familial ties. The emphasis on positive reinforcement, effective communication, collaborative problem-solving, and collective self-care creates a foundation upon which recovery can be built and sustained.

4.3 Utilizing MI Techniques in Family Conversations

Motivational Interviewing (MI), with its roots in counseling, offers a nuanced approach to communication that can be a lifeline for families navigating the complexities of addiction. It's not just about talking; it's about connecting in ways that foster trust, understanding, and a genuine desire for change. This section explores how families can employ MI techniques to engage their loved ones in meaningful dialogue about recovery, enhancing motivation, and respecting the individual's journey toward change.

Engaging the Loved One:

Opening a dialogue with a loved one about addiction and recovery is akin to navigating a minefield. The fear of stepping wrong and triggering an explosion of defensiveness or denial is palpable. Here, the essence of MI—emphasizing empathy and acceptance—becomes invaluable. It involves:

- Initiating conversations with an open heart, ready to listen more than speak. It's about creating a safe space for sharing fears and hopes without judgment.
- Posing open-ended questions, encouraging the loved one to express their thoughts and feelings in their own words. These questions should invite elaboration, not just yes or no answers.
- Reflecting what you hear, not as a parrot would, but with an interpretation that shows you're trying to understand the depth of their experience. This reflection also checks your understanding and corrects any misinterpretations.

These techniques gently invite the loved one into a conversation, making it easier for them to open up and share their perspectives.

Expressing Empathy through Reflection

Empathy, the ability to understand and share the feelings of another is the cornerstone of MI and a powerful tool in family conversations. Reflective listening, where you mirror back the emotions and meanings you hear in your loved one's words, demonstrates empathy in action. This process:

- Validates the loved one's feelings, showing them that their experiences and emotions are understood and accepted.
- Helps to lower walls of defensiveness, fostering a climate where open, honest dialogue can flourish.
- Encourages deeper exploration of the issues, often revealing underlying concerns or desires that somebody might not have voiced otherwise.

Through reflective listening, families can create a dialogue that feels more like a bridge than a barrier, connecting them to their shared experience.

Enhancing Motivation for Change

At the heart of MI is the recognition that the motivation for change must come from within. For families, this means inspiring their loved ones to consider change, not through coercion or persuasion, but by exploring the discrepancies between their current behaviors and their deeper values or life goals. This exploration can be facilitated by

- Gently pointing out contradictions between the loved one's actions and their stated desires or values in a curious rather than accusatory way. It's about asking questions that help them see these discrepancies for themselves.
- Focusing on past successes and strengths, reminding the loved one of their capabilities and potential. This focus builds confidence in their ability to change.
- Discussing the future, exploring how different choices might lead to different outcomes. This conversation is framed around hope and possibility, not fear.

By nurturing motivation in this way, families can support their loved ones in finding reasons to pursue recovery that resonate with their values and aspirations.

Respecting Autonomy

A fundamental principle of MI is the respect for the individual's autonomy, their right to make their own choices. For families, this means shifting from a directive approach to supporting the loved one's sense of agency and control over their recovery journey. This approach involves

- Offering information and support but allowing the loved one to decide what steps to take. It's about being a partner in the process, not the director.
- Encouraging the development of self-efficacy, the belief in one's ability to effect change. Self-efficacy might involve highlighting past instances where the loved one successfully navigated challenges or made positive choices.
- Recognizing and respecting the loved one's right to make decisions, even those the family might disagree with. It's about offering guidance and support, not ultimatums.

By respecting autonomy, families can foster a sense of empowerment in their loved ones, a critical component in the journey toward recovery.

In weaving MI techniques into family conversations, a transformation occurs. Dialogue becomes a tool for communication, connection, understanding, and growth. It's a shift from confrontation to collaboration, where every conversation can bring the family closer to healing and the loved one closer to recovery. Through empathy, motivation, and respect, families can navigate the complexities of addiction with compassion and hope, supporting their loved ones in finding their path toward change.

4.4 Applying ACT in the Context of Family Addiction

Understanding and Acceptance

In the heart of Acceptance and Commitment Therapy (ACT) lies a profound lesson for families: addiction, as daunting as it may seem, is a condition that thrives in the shadows of misunderstanding and stigma. Families are invited to cultivate a deep understanding and acceptance of addiction. This doesn't mean resigning to it but acknowledging its presence without judgment. Through this lens, the condition is seen not as a series of failed choices but as a complex interplay of factors beyond one's control.

To foster this understanding, families can

- Engage in open dialogues about the realities of addiction, emphasizing its medical and psychological aspects.
- Practice empathy by imagining the world from the perspective of their loved one, understanding their fears, challenges, and the weight of addiction on their shoulders.
- Educate themselves about the myths surrounding addiction, actively seeking information from reliable sources to dismantle preconceived notions.

This path towards understanding and acceptance is the first step in changing the family's narrative around addiction, paving the way for a more compassionate and supportive environment.

Mindfulness Practices

Stress and anxiety are frequent travelers on the road of addiction recovery for both the individual and their family members. Mindfulness practices offer a refuge, a momentary pause where the mind and body can find equilibrium. By focusing on the present, families can break free from the cycle of worry about the future and regrets about the past, reducing overall stress levels.

Mindfulness can be woven into family life through

- Daily mindfulness moments where family members spend a few minutes in silence, focusing on their breath or a simple meditation.
- Mindful eating exercises during family meals focus on the experience of eating, the flavors, textures, and the act of nourishment.
- Nature walks where the family observes their surroundings, focusing on the sights, sounds, and smells, grounding themselves in the present moment.

These practices reduce stress and anxiety and enhance the family's ability to communicate and support each other with patience and understanding.

Values-Driven Actions

ACT emphasizes living by one's values, a principle that can significantly impact families dealing with addiction. By identifying and embracing these core values, families can navigate the recovery process with clarity and purpose, ensuring their actions and decisions support their loved one's recovery and the family's overall well-being.

To identify and act on these values, families can:

- Hold a family meeting to discuss and identify their collective values, such as honesty, compassion, or resilience.
- Set goals based on these values, creating actionable steps that embody these principles in daily life.
- Regularly reflect on these actions, assessing whether they align with the family's values and making adjustments as needed.

Living in alignment with shared values fosters a sense of unity and purpose, guiding the family through the challenges of addiction with integrity and strength.

Commitment to Change

The journey through addiction is marked by change, requiring a commitment from both the individual and their family. ACT's principle of commitment encourages families to pledge to support recovery, embracing the necessary changes within the family dynamics that promote healing and growth. This commitment isn't static; it evolves, adapting to the challenges and successes.

Families can manifest this commitment by

- Creating a recovery plan that includes specific roles and responsibilities for each family member, ensuring everyone is actively involved.

- Establish rituals reinforcing the family's commitment to recovery, such as weekly check-ins or celebrating milestones.
- Being open to revisiting and revising the commitment as the family navigates through the recovery process, ensuring it remains relevant and supportive.

This proactive stance on change strengthens the family's resilience, empowering them to face the ups and downs of recovery with confidence and unity.

As we close this exploration of Acceptance and Commitment Therapy within the realm of family addiction, the core themes of understanding, mindfulness, values-driven actions, and commitment weave together to form a tapestry of support. These principles guide families in creating an environment where recovery is not just a possibility but a shared journey embraced with empathy, patience, and purpose. Moving forward, the emphasis shifts to sustaining these efforts, ensuring the family remains a pillar of strength and support for their loved one on the path to recovery.

CHAPTER 5
SUSTAINING THE MOMENTUM OF RECOVERY

The road to recovery is paved with the bricks of support, understanding, and love. Each step taken is a testament to the resilience not just of the individual in recovery but of their entire family network. However, the true challenge lies not in taking the first step, but in keeping the pace, ensuring each foot is placed with as much intention as the last. The journey does not end with sobriety; it merely shifts gears, moving from the rugged terrain of overcoming addiction to the winding paths of maintaining it. Here, the emphasis shifts towards the support networks that act as the guardrails, keeping the individual on track, and the family unit cohesive and strong.

5.1 Community and Connection

The significance of a robust support network can't be overstated. Picture a tree, its branches spreading wide, offering shade and shelter. This tree, however, is only as sturdy as the root system below. Similarly, the recovery process leans heavily on the roots established through community connections, support groups, and sober networks. These roots provide the necessary nutrients—advice, empathy, understanding—feeding the individual's resolve to stay on the path of recovery.

- Support groups like Alcoholics Anonymous or Narcotics Anonymous offer a space where individuals can share their experiences without fear of judgment, drawing strength from the collective wisdom of those who've walked similar paths.
- Sober networks, often formed within rehabilitation programs or local community centers, consist of individuals committed to living a substance-free life. Engaging in activities, from hiking to coffee meetups, reinforces the lifestyle changes integral to recovery.
- Online communities also play a crucial role, especially in remote areas. Websites and social media platforms dedicated to recovery provide access to resources, inspirational stories, and 24/7 support from peers worldwide.

For families, actively participating in these networks alongside their loved ones reinforces unity and shows a collective commitment to recovery. It's about showing up, whether by attending open meetings or supporting and organizing sober activities.

Family Engagement

The family's role evolves as recovery progresses. Initially, the focus might be crisis management and getting through each day. As recovery becomes more stable, the approach shifts towards positive reinforcement and shared experiences that support sobriety.

- Positive reinforcement involves acknowledging and celebrating the milestones, no matter how small. It's about noticing and appreciating the efforts towards sobriety, from attending meetings to being more present during family time.
- Shared activities that promote sobriety and wellness are crucial. This could be a weekly family hike, cooking healthy meals together, or taking up a new hobby as a family. These activities strengthen the bond and support the lifestyle changes critical to long-term recovery.

Professional Support

Continued engagement with addiction professionals, therapists, and counselors ensures the family and the individual have access to expert guidance tailored to the evolving challenges of recovery.

- Regular check-ins with a therapist can help the individual in recovery navigate the complexities of life post-addiction, offering strategies to manage stress, triggers, and the inevitable bumps along the road.
- Family therapy sessions remain invaluable, providing a space to address ongoing dynamics, communication challenges, and emerging issues in a supportive, mediated environment.

Peer Support

Engaging in peer support roles offers individuals in recovery a unique opportunity to reinforce their sobriety while contributing to the recovery of others. This reciprocal, rel-cultivating self-esteem provides a sense of purpose and strengthens the commitment to sobriety.

- Mentoring or sponsorship within support groups benefits those new to recovery and solidifies the mentor's resolve and understanding of the recovery process.
- Volunteering at local recovery centers or community events related to sobriety and wellness allows individuals to give back, creating a positive feedback loop that bolsters their and others' journeys.

Sustaining recovery is an ongoing process, requiring dedication, adaptability, and a strong support network. Through community connections, family engagement, professional guidance, and peer support, the path to long-term sobriety becomes a possibility and a reality, paved with the collective efforts and commitment of all involved.

5.2 Adapting to Life Post-Addiction

Recovery reshapes the landscape of daily life, introducing a new rhythm to the once-familiar melody of family routines, relationships, and social engagements. This adjustment period, while challenging, opens doors to a revitalized way of living that prioritizes health, connection, and growth.

New Normals

In this transition, families redefine what 'normal' looks like. This redefinition isn't just about adapting to the absence of substances but about reimagining the fabric of family life to support sustained well-being.

- Redefining family roles becomes necessary as each member explores new dynamics free from the constraints of addiction. Open discussions can help redistribute responsibilities and expectations, allowing for a more balanced and supportive household.
- Revisiting traditions and routines is crucial. Simple adjustments, replacing a routine that may have centered around substance use with new traditions like family game nights or morning walks, can reinforce a sense of unity and shared commitment to a healthier lifestyle.
- Reinforcing positive changes with daily affirmations or a visual board can help the family stay aligned with their new routine, celebrating the progress and reminding everyone of the shared vision for the future.

Healthy Lifestyle Choices

A cornerstone of lasting recovery is cultivating healthy habits that support physical and emotional well-being.

- Encouraging regular physical activity is vital. Whether it's group sports, individual fitness goals, or family hikes, staying active boosts mood, improves health, and strengthens bonds.

- Prioritizing nutrition involves more than just healthy eating; it's about making meal preparation a shared family activity that values nourishment and togetherness.
- Implementing stress management techniques, from mindfulness meditation to breathing exercises, can be a collective endeavor, enhancing the family's capacity to navigate stress healthily.

Navigating Social Situations

Social environments present complex challenges for those in recovery, laden with potential triggers and pressure, while providing a pivotal role in navigating these waters.

- Preparing a plan before attending social events can empower individuals in recovery, offering them a sense of control and readiness to face potential challenges. This plan might include a code word for when they feel uncomfortable and need to leave or a list of non-alcoholic drinks they can enjoy.
- Setting boundaries around social engagements is essential. This might mean choosing events that align with recovery goals or declining invitations to environments that pose too high a risk.
- Having an exit strategy is not about running away; it's about knowing when to step back to protect one's progress. Leaving an event early or having a trusted family member on call ensures safety without sacrificing a social life.

Embracing Growth and Change

The post-addiction phase is ripe with opportunities for personal development and family growth. Embracing this period as a transformation can invigorate the family unit with renewed purpose and direction.

- Encouraging individual pursuits, such as hobbies, education, or career goals, supports personal growth and self-esteem. Celebrating these achievements as a family reinforces the value of each member's journey.
- Engaging in collective goals or projects, whether a family garden, a community service project, or a shared learning endeavor, fosters a sense of teamwork and shared purpose.
- Fostering open communication about the changes and challenges reinforces the family's resilience. It's about creating a safe space where feelings of uncertainty, fear, or excitement can be shared and navigated together.

In adapting to life post-addiction, families traverse a landscape marked by change. Yet, within this terrain lie opportunities to rebuild stronger, more connected, and healthier than before. The journey may be continuous, but each step forward is a step towards a future brimming with possibility.

5.3 Preventing Burnout in Caregivers

Caring for a loved one navigating the path of recovery from addiction is akin to tending a garden that requires constant nurturing, patience, and understanding. While admirable and filled with love, this dedication often comes with its own challenges, notably the risk of caregiver burnout. Recognizing the early signs of this burnout, building resilience, seeking help, and ensuring responsibilities are shared are not just acts of self-preservation but are crucial for the continued support of the individual in recovery.

Recognizing the Signs

Burnout creeps in silently, often mistaken for mere tiredness or a bad day. However, its markers are distinct—a pervasive sense of fatigue that rest doesn't cure, irritability over minor inconveniences, and a feeling of detachment or reduced personal accomplishment in caregiving roles. Physical manifestations might include headaches, stomachaches, or a change in appetite. Emotional signs could manifest as sadness, anxiety, or a feeling of hopelessness. In recognizing these signs early, families can take proactive steps to address them, preventing further escalation that could impair their ability to provide care.

Building Resilience

Resilience in caregivers is like the roots of a tree, allowing it to bend in the storm but not break. Developing this resilience involves several vital strategies:

- Cultivating a solid support network that is not limited to those directly involved in the caregiving. This network might include friends, relatives, or members of support groups who can offer emotional backing and practical assistance.
- Regular self-care activities are fundamental. Engaging in hobbies that bring joy, exercising to relieve stress,

or simply allowing time for relaxation can replenish a caregiver's emotional and physical energy.

- Setting realistic expectations for the recovery process helps mitigate disappointment or failure. Understanding that recovery is a nonlinear process with potential setbacks can temper frustrations and foster a more patient, supportive approach.

These strategies fortify caregivers against the pressures associated with their role and enhance their overall well-being, ensuring they remain a steadfast pillar of support for their loved ones.

Seeking Help

The act of reaching out for help is a strength, not a weakness. It recognizes the caregiver's needs and is a crucial step in safeguarding their health. Various avenues for assistance include:

- Therapy or counseling can offer a space to explore and process the complex emotions associated with caregiving, providing coping strategies and emotional support.
- Support groups designed for caregivers offer a sense of community, understanding, and shared experiences, reducing feelings of isolation.
- Respite care gives caregivers a temporary break, allowing them time to recharge. This can be through professional services or by enlisting the help of friends and family for short periods.

These resources offer relief and ensure caregivers have access to the emotional and practical support necessary to continue their caregiving journey without compromising their own well-being.

Shared Responsibility

The proverb "It takes a village to raise a child" holds in the context of caregiving during recovery. Distributing care responsibilities among multiple family members and friends prevents the concentration of burden on a single individual, promoting a more sustainable support system. This distribution might look like this:

- Rotating schedules among family and friends to ensure the caregiver has regular breaks.
- Assigning specific tasks based on individual strengths or availability, such as one person handling appointments while another focuses on daily physical activities with the loved one.
- Open communication about the needs and limits of each support member to ensure tasks are manageable and within their capability.

This approach alleviates the pressure on the primary caregiver. It fosters a collective effort to support the loved one's recovery, reinforcing the idea that a community of care and support surrounds them.

In navigating the multifaceted roles of caregiving, families must remain vigilant to the signs of burnout, actively seek ways to build resilience, reach out for help when needed, and embrace the concept of shared responsibility. These steps ensure that caregivers can sustain their support for their loved ones in recovery without sacrificing their health and happiness. This balance is crucial, not just for the individual's well-being in recovery but for the holistic health of the family unit, ensuring every member, caregiver included, is nurtured and supported through this journey.

5.4 Continuing Education and Growth

In recovery, education stretches beyond the conventional classroom. It becomes a vibrant, ongoing process where families and those in recovery immerse themselves in learning not just about the nuances of addiction but about the myriad ways to foster personal development and resilience. This commitment to learning serves as a beacon, guiding each step with informed choices and a deeper understanding of the recovery landscape.

Lifelong Learning

The path of recovery introduces a landscape rich with lessons on human strength, vulnerability, and the capacity for change. Families find themselves in a continuous loop of learning, where each day offers insights into the complexities of addiction and the resilience of the human spirit. This educational journey can take many forms:

- Attending workshops and seminars becomes a way to stay informed about the latest research and strategies in addiction recovery.
- Reading books and articles broadens horizons, offering new perspectives and coping strategies.
- Participating in online courses or webinars allows families to deepen their understanding of

psychological principles and therapeutic approaches that underpin successful recovery.

This commitment to ongoing education ensures that families remain equipped with the knowledge to support their loved ones effectively, adapting to challenges with insight and understanding.

Adapting Strategies Over Time

As the seasons change, so do the needs of individuals in recovery and their families. What works at the onset of recovery might not hold the same efficacy. This fluidity requires an open-minded approach to adapting strategies, ensuring they align with the evolving recovery journey. Considerations include:

- Staying abreast of emerging therapies and support mechanisms that might offer new avenues for growth and healing.
- Reflecting on the efficacy of current strategies and being willing to pivot as needed, whether that means exploring new therapeutic modalities or adjusting support structures within the family.
- Encouraging feedback from the individual in recovery about what is helping or hindering their progress, fostering a collaborative approach to adjusting strategies.

Embracing change in this way keeps the recovery process dynamic, responsive, and attuned to each individual's unique path.

Engaging in New Activities

The tapestry of recovery is woven with threads of new experiences and challenges. Engaging in new activities and hobbies offers a canvas for individuals in recovery and their families to paint their journeys with vibrant colors of joy, learning, and connection. These activities:

- Provide opportunities for developing new skills and interests, contributing to a sense of accomplishment and self-esteem.
- Offer a constructive outlet for energy and emotions as a valuable tool for managing stress and preventing relapse.
- Facilitate positive social interactions, helping to rebuild the social confidence that addiction may have eroded.

From art classes to hiking clubs, these new pursuits enrich the recovery experience, bringing light and texture to the healing journey.

Fostering a Growth Mindset

At the heart of ongoing education and adaptation lies the cultivation of a growth mindset—a belief in the potential for continuous improvement and learning from all experiences. This mindset encourages families and individuals in recovery to

- View challenges as opportunities for growth rather than insurmountable obstacles.

- Celebrate progress, however small, recognizing each step forward as a victory.
- Embrace setbacks as learning opportunities, analyzing what went awry and how to adjust.

This perspective transforms the recovery process into an expansive journey of self-discovery and development, where every moment holds growth potential.

As we wrap up this exploration of continuing education and growth, it's clear that the path of recovery is not static but a vibrant journey marked by constant learning and adaptation. By committing to lifelong learning, staying flexible in the face of change, exploring new activities, and embracing a growth mindset, families and individuals in recovery can navigate the twists and turns with resilience and hope. This approach not only supports the immediate goals of recovery but also lays a foundation for a fulfilling life, rich with possibilities and new horizons.

As we move forward, let us carry the lessons learned and the knowledge gained, ready to face the challenges and opportunities ahead with courage, compassion, and an unwavering commitment to growth.

CHAPTER 6
BUILDING A FUTURE TOGETHER

Imagine standing at the edge of a vast, beautiful landscape stretching far and wide. Ahead lies a winding path filled with unknowns yet promising growth, healing, and unity. This is where families, having navigated the tumultuous waters of addiction, find themselves as they look toward a life beyond addiction. It's about piecing together a shared vision, setting goals, celebrating progress, and staying flexible as life unfolds.

6.1 Creating a Shared Vision

Crafting a shared vision is like painting a family portrait, where each member's hopes, dreams, and aspirations are the colors that bring the picture to life. This vision acts as a north star, guiding decisions and actions.

- **Family Meetings:** Regular sit-downs allow everyone to voice their thoughts on what they envision for the future. It's a collaborative effort, blending individual hopes into a collective aspiration.

- **Vision Board:** Visuals can be powerful. Creating a physical or digital board filled with images, quotes, and symbols representing the family's shared goals can be a daily reminder of what you're all working towards.
- **Open Communication:** Ensuring every voice is heard and valued is vital. This means active listening and acknowledging different perspectives, even when they diverge.

Setting Achievable Goals

Goals are the steps leading towards the vision. They turn the abstract into something tangible, something you can reach out and touch.

- **Short-term Milestones:** These are immediate goals that feel attainable, like attending weekly family therapy sessions or organizing a monthly family outing. Celebrating these can boost morale and motivation.
- **Long-term Objectives:** These are the broader aims, perhaps financial stability or a healthier lifestyle. They require patience and persistence, often involving smaller steps that accumulate over time.
- **Regular Reviews:** Life changes, and so do goals. Regularly checking in on these goals allows you to adjust and realign as needed.

Celebrating Progress

Every step forward deserves recognition. It's not just about the big wins but also the tiny victories that often go unnoticed.

- **Acknowledgment:** Simple acknowledgments, such as verbal praises during family dinners or notes of encouragement, can uplift spirits.
- **Celebration Rituals:** Establishing rituals, like a special dinner for milestones or a family movie night after a week of achievements, adds joy and anticipation to the journey of progress.
- **Recording Success:** Keeping a journal or a digital log of achievements helps track progress and reminds you how far you've come, especially during challenging times.

Adjusting Expectations

Flexibility is the compass that helps navigate the unpredictable nature of life and recovery. It's about bending, not breaking, under the pressures of unexpected changes.

- **Open Dialogues on Change:** When life throws a curveball, openly discussing how this impacts your goals and vision is crucial. It ensures everyone is on the same page and can adjust their sails accordingly.
- **Embrace Learning:** Every misstep or detour is a learning opportunity. It's about finding the lesson in every situation and using it to strengthen your resolve and approach.

- **Support System:** Leaning on external supports, such as therapy groups or friends, provides perspective and guidance during times of change.

This chapter opens doors to a hopeful future, where families, having weathered the storm of addiction, can now navigate the calm and sometimes uncertain waters that lie ahead. It's a testament to the power of unity, resilience, and love in building a life filled with possibilities and joy.

Collaborative Goal Setting

goals within a family should be a collective endeavor where everyone's voice has weight and significance. This process nurtures a sense of unity as each member contributes to the tapestry of shared aspirations.

- Initiate a 'Goal-setting Day,' making it a special occasion on the family calendar. This day is dedicated to discussing and outlining the goals for the upcoming months or years. Ensure this is an enjoyable experience, perhaps by preparing a favorite family meal or incorporating a fun post-discussion activity.
- Use a large sheet of paper or a whiteboard to map the goals visually. This visual representation can be a powerful tool, making the abstract more tangible. Each family member can write or draw their goals, explaining their significance to the rest.
- Emphasize the importance of listening during this process. It's not just about speaking up but also about appreciating the perspectives and aspirations of others. This ensures that everyone feels heard and

valued, reinforcing the bond between family members.

Balancing Individual and Collective Goals

In a family, especially one navigating the waters of addiction recovery, the harmony between individual and collective goals is crucial. It's about finding the delicate balance for personal growth while fostering family unity.

- For individual goals, particularly those of the family member in recovery, it's vital to ensure these are realistic and aligned with their recovery process. These might include attending support meetings regularly or pursuing a hobby that brings joy and fulfillment.
- Collective goals could range from improving communication within the family to planning a family vacation. These goals mustn't overshadow the individual goals of the recovering member but instead complement them, creating an environment where personal achievements and family milestones are celebrated with equal enthusiasm.
- Regular check-ins can help maintain this balance. These are opportunities to assess how well individual and collective goals are being met and whether one set takes precedence over the other, allowing for real-time adjustments.

Integrating New Traditions and Rituals

Traditions and rituals, old and new, are the glue that binds a family together, offering a sense of identity and belonging. In recovery, introducing new traditions can symbolize the family's evolution and a renewed commitment to each other's well-being.

- Consider traditions that promote health and well-being, such as a weekly family hike or a monthly 'unplugged' day where all electronic devices are set aside in favor of outdoor activities or board games.
- Rituals can also be small, everyday habits that build connection, like sharing one thing you're grateful for at dinner or a morning hug. These acts, though simple, can significantly impact the family's emotional climate.
- Allow these traditions and rituals to evolve organically. What starts as a one-time activity could naturally become a cherished family custom, reflecting the family's growth and changing dynamics.

Monitoring and Revising Goals

The path to achieving goals is rarely linear. It twists and turns, presenting unforeseen challenges and opportunities for growth. Regularly monitoring progress and being willing to revise goals accordingly is a testament to the family's adaptability and commitment to their shared vision.

- Set aside a time each month for a goal review session. This is a chance to celebrate small successes and address any areas where progress may be lagging. It's also an opportunity to reassess the relevance of each goal, ensuring they still align with the family's vision and circumstances.

- Encourage transparency during these reviews. If a goal proves too challenging, this is the time to speak up. Perhaps the goal needs to be broken down into smaller, more manageable steps, or maybe it's no longer relevant and should be replaced.
- Remember, revising goals is not a sign of failure but of flexibility and resilience. It reflects the family's ability to navigate change, making adjustments that keep them on track toward their shared vision.

Families forge a more profound connection in this continuous cycle of setting, pursuing, and revisiting goals. They learn the art of compromise, the strength in unity, and the joy of celebrating each step forward together. While not always easy, this process is rich with opportunities for growth, healing, and creating a future filled with hope and possibility.

6.2 The Role of Community in Recovery

In the landscape of recovery, the fabric of family support is undeniably crucial, yet the weave of community involvement adds both strength and texture that enriches the recovery process. This section explores the multifaceted role of the community in recovery, emphasizing the expansion of the support network, the transformative power of community service, the learning opportunities from diverse experiences, and the potential to create a legacy of hope.

Expanding the Support Network

The support network for a family and their loved one in recovery can significantly benefit from branching out beyond the immediate circle of close friends and family. This expansion involves

- Identifying and engaging with local organizations focused on recovery and mental health support. These groups often offer workshops, counseling, and social events that can provide additional support layers.
- Embracing support groups specific to the family's needs. For instance, groups for parents, spouses, or siblings of those in recovery can offer targeted advice and shared experiences that resonate more deeply with each family member's unique perspective.
- Leveraging online platforms for support. Many online communities provide 24/7 access to resources and peer support, which can be invaluable, especially when local groups are not meeting or when privacy concerns prevent someone from reaching out in person.

Expanding the support network is akin to casting a wider net. It ensures that the family and the individual in recovery have access to various resources, advice, and emotional support that can adapt to their evolving needs.

Community Service and Engagement

Participation in community service projects presents a unique avenue for individuals in recovery and their families to step outside their personal experiences, offering their time and energy to causes that benefit the wider community. This engagement can

- Foster a sense of purpose and self-worth, reminding individuals in recovery that they have valuable contributions to make.
- Build new social connections with those outside the immediate circle of recovery support, offering fresh perspectives and reducing the sense of isolation that often accompanies addiction.
- Provide practical experiences that can enhance personal growth, such as teamwork, leadership, and communication skills.

Whether volunteering at a local food bank, participating in environmental cleanup projects, or organizing fundraising events for local charities, community service is a reciprocal process. It enriches both the giver and the receiver, embedding the individual and their family within a network of positive social change.

Learning from Diverse Experiences

The recovery community is a tapestry of stories, each thread colored by unique experiences and insights. Families can deepen their understanding and broaden their perspectives on recovery by:

- Attending open meetings and workshops where stories of addiction and recovery are shared. These narratives can offer hope, inspiration, and practical strategies that families might not encounter in their immediate circles.
- Participating in educational events hosted by recovery organizations or health services. These events often cover the latest research in addiction

science, treatment modalities, and holistic approaches to wellness.

- Encouraging dialogues with individuals from different backgrounds and stages of recovery. These conversations can challenge preconceptions, illuminate the diverse paths of recovery, and foster a more inclusive approach to supporting their loved ones.

By actively seeking out and embracing these diverse experiences, families can equip themselves with a richer, more nuanced understanding of recovery. This knowledge not only aids in navigating their loved one's recovery process but also prepares them to offer informed support to others embarking on similar paths.

Building a Legacy of Hope

The journey from addiction to recovery is fraught with challenges, yet it also offers the unparalleled opportunity to forge a legacy of hope and resilience. Families can transform their experiences into beacons for others by

- Sharing their stories through community talks, blogs, or social media. Openly discussing the struggles and triumphs of their journey can offer solace and guidance to others feeling lost in the mire of addiction.
- Creating or participating in support initiatives that address gaps they may have encountered. This could involve setting up scholarship funds for recovery programs, launching awareness campaigns, or

advocating for policy changes related to addiction and mental health.

- Mentoring other families new to the recovery process. Providing a listening ear, practical advice, or simply being a presence that says, "You are not alone," can make a monumental difference in the lives of those just beginning to navigate these waters.

Through these actions, families contribute to the healing and growth of their communities and cement a legacy that transcends their personal journey. It's a testament to the power of shared experiences, the strength found in communal support, and the enduring light of hope that guides the way forward for all touched by addiction.

6.3 A Toolkit for Resilience and Hope

Navigating the path of recovery requires more than just a map; it demands a toolkit equipped with the right resources, strategies, and practices. This toolkit becomes a lifeline for families and individuals, enabling them to maintain the momentum of recovery, build resilience, and keep hope alive. It's a collection of practical aids drawn from the wealth of insights shared in our discussions, tailored to meet the unique challenges and triumphs that mark the recovery landscape.

Essential Tools for Sustaining Recovery

At the heart of this toolkit are essential resources designed to support the individual and their family in recovery. These tools are not merely aids but are the building blocks for a foundation strong enough to support the weight of recovery and flexible sufficient to adapt to its ebbs and flows. They include

- A list of local and online support groups that offer a sense of community and understanding. These groups provide a space where experiences are shared and encouragement is abundant.
- A collection of mindfulness and stress-reduction techniques, from simple breathing exercises to structured meditation practices. These techniques are vital for managing the stresses that inevitably accompany recovery.
- A journal for tracking progress, thoughts, and feelings. This can be a powerful tool for reflection and growth, offering a tangible record of the journey and the milestones.
- Educational materials on addiction and recovery, including books, articles, and websites. Knowledge empowers families, enabling them to navigate recovery with confidence and compassion.
- A plan for healthy living, incorporating physical activity, nutrition, and sleep. Wellness in these areas supports overall recovery, providing the energy and strength needed to face challenges.

Customizing the Toolkit

While the foundation of the toolkit is universal, its true strength lies in its ability to be customized. Each family each individual in recovery, brings their own story and needs to the table. Customizing the toolkit involves:

- Identifying the strategies that resonate most with the individual and family. What works for one may not work for another, and that's okay. It's about finding the right fit.
- Incorporating personal goals into the toolkit. Whether it's rebuilding relationships, pursuing new hobbies, or furthering education, these goals are the personal touches that make the toolkit genuinely effective.
- Regularly review and update the toolkit to reflect changes in circumstances, challenges, and achievements. Flexibility ensures that the toolkit remains relevant and practical.

Sharing the Toolkit

The power of the toolkit is not just in its use but in its potential to inspire and support others in the recovery community. Sharing the toolkit can take many forms:

- Offering copies of the journal, complete with reflections and progress, to others beginning their recovery journey. This can provide hope and a sense of what's possible.
- Hosting workshops or discussion groups based on the educational materials that have been most impactful. This reinforces the family's learning and extends that knowledge to others.
- Sharing lists of resources, from support groups to stress-reduction techniques, with online communities or local recovery organizations. This sharing is a ripple effect, extending support beyond the immediate circle.

Continued Evolution

Like the path of recovery itself, the toolkit is dynamic. It evolves, shifts, and grows in response to discoveries, challenges, and victories. Its evolution is marked by:

- The integration of new resources and strategies as they are discovered. Recovery is a field continually enriched by research and personal experiences, offering fresh insights that can enhance the toolkit.
- The adaptation to meet new phases of recovery. As individuals and families grow, their needs change. The toolkit must change with them, reflecting the journey's current landscape.
- Celebrations of achievements, both big and small. Each victory, each hurdle overcome, is a testament to resilience and hope, reinforcing the value of the toolkit and the efforts invested in recovery.

In closing, this toolkit is a testament to the strength, courage, and love families and individuals bring to the recovery process. It's a collection of resources, a compilation of strategies, and a repository of hope designed to support, guide, and inspire. As we move forward, let us carry the lessons learned, the tools discovered, and the hope kindled, ready to face the challenges and opportunities ahead with resilience and optimism.

CONCLUSION

As we draw this journey to a close—a journey that has taken us through the intricate landscapes of understanding addiction, resilience in the face of adversity, and the empowerment that comes from applying evidence-based strategies—I want to acknowledge the steps you've taken just by engaging with the pages of this book. From grappling with the multifaceted nature of addiction and its ripple effects on the family system to embracing the practice of setting healthy boundaries and employing strategies like CRAFT, MI, and ACT, you've embarked on a path not just to support your loved one, but to transform and enrich your family dynamics in profound ways.

Empathy and compassion have been our guiding lights, illuminating the importance of approaching your loved one and yourself with understanding and kindness. These are soft virtues and powerful tools that create an environment where healing and recovery can flourish.

The emphasis on self-care for caregivers cannot be overstated. Remember, caring for yourself is not an act of selfishness but a necessity. It's the oxygen mask principle—you must be well to support those around you effectively. This book has aimed to underscore that taking care of your well-being allows you to be the pillar of strength your loved one needs on their journey to recovery.

The strategies we've delved into—CRAFT, MI, and ACT—have been demystified and presented as accessible tools that you, as a family, can wield to navigate addiction challenges. These approaches empower you with practical methods to support your loved one while fostering hope and delineating a concrete path toward a healthier future.

Recovery, as we've explored, is an ongoing journey marked by its ups and downs. It's a path of continuous effort, learning, and support that doesn't end at a specific destination. I encourage you to view setbacks not as failures but as integral steps in growth and healing.

Building a supportive community extends beyond the confines of your immediate family. Engaging with support groups and therapists and leveraging community resources can bolster your resilience and provide a broader safety net for you and your loved one. This support network is invaluable, offering different perspectives, shared experiences, and additional strength to draw upon.

I urge you to take the strategies and insights gleaned from our time together and actively apply them in your lives. Share your journey, challenges, and victories, no matter how small, with others who might be navigating similar tumultuous waters. In doing so, you contribute to a broader community of support, understanding, and compassion.

As you continue on this path, hold onto hope and encouragement. The road to recovery is challenging and filled with moments that test your resolve, patience, and strength. Yet, it is also a journey punctuated with opportunities for incredible growth, deeper connections, and healing. You are not walking this path alone. Change is possible, and with love, perseverance, and applying the strategies we've discussed, a brighter future lies ahead.

For those seeking further guidance, support, or resources, remember that help is always available. Whether through websites dedicated to addiction recovery, directories of support groups, or a list of recommended readings, there are avenues open to you for continued support beyond these pages.

I want to express my gratitude for allowing me to join your journey. Together, we've explored the depths of a complex issue, believing that understanding, empathy, and informed action can pave the way for recovery and renewal. Keep moving forward, one step at a time, with the knowledge that each day brings new opportunities for healing and hope.

With warmest regards and encouragement,
Jeremy

REFERENCES

- *Traumatic Stress and Substance Abuse Problems* https://istss.org/ISTSS_Main/media/Documents/ISTSS_TraumaStressandSubstanceAbuseProb_English_FNL.pdf
- *The Science of Addiction Treatment and Recovery* https://nida.nih.gov/publications/drugs-brains-behavior-science-addiction/treatment-recovery
- *The Role Of Family In Addiction Recovery* https://www.addictioncenter.com/addiction/role-family-addiction-recovery/
- *Intervention: Help a loved one overcome addiction* https://www.mayoclinic.org/diseases-conditions/mental-illness/in-depth/intervention/art-20047451
- *Setting Boundaries With An Addict | 7 Ways To Start* https://peaksrecovery.com/blog/other/setting-appropriate-boundaries-with-an-addict/
- *The Importance of Communication Skills in Recovery* https://www.ashleytreatment.org/rehab-blog/the-importance-of-communication-skills-in-recovery/
- *The Impact of Substance Use Disorders on Families and ...* https://www.ncbi.nlm.nih.gov/pmc/articles/PMC3725219/
- *Self-Care For Family And Friends Of People With Addiction* https://theridgeohio.com/blog/self-care/
- *Chapter 3—Family Counseling Approaches* https://www.ncbi.nlm.nih.gov/books/NBK571088/
- *Caregiver Burnout: What It Is, Symptoms & Prevention* https://my.clevelandclinic.org/health/diseases/9225-caregiver-burnout
- *SAMHSA's National Helpline* https://www.samhsa.gov/find-help/national-helpline

- *Drug Rehab vs. Detox: What is the Difference?* https://www.turnbridge.com/news-events/latest-articles/drug-rehab-vs-detox/

- *The CRAFT Approach to Substance Abuse Intervention* https://www.verywellmind.com/the-craft-approach-to-substance-abuse-intervention-5191125

- *USING MOTIVATIONAL INTERVIEWING IN - Advisory 35* https://store.samhsa.gov/sites/default/files/PEP20-02-02-014.pdf

- *What is Acceptance and Commitment Therapy (ACT) ...* https://createbehaviorsolutions.com/what-is-acceptance-and-commitment-therapy-act-and-why-it-is-useful-for-parents/

- *TIP 39 Substance Use Disorder Treatment and Family ...* https://store.samhsa.gov/sites/default/files/tip-39-treatment-family-therapy-pep20-02-02-012.pdf

- *Benefits of peer support groups in the treatment of addiction* https://www.ncbi.nlm.nih.gov/pmc/articles/PMC5047716/

- *Caregiver stress: Tips for taking care of yourself - Mayo Clinic* https://www.mayoclinic.org/healthy-lifestyle/stress-management/in-depth/caregiver-stress/art-20044784

- *Tips For Staying Sober: Navigating Social Situations While ...* https://quest2recovery.com/blog/staying-sober/

- *Impact of Continuing Care on Recovery From Substance ...* https://www.ncbi.nlm.nih.gov/pmc/articles/PMC7813220/

- *Setting SMART Goals in Recovery* https://www.ashleytreatment.org/rehab-blog/setting-smart-goals-in-recovery/

- *The Importance of Community In Recovery* https://journeypureriver.com/importance-community-recovery/

- *Creating New Sober Holiday Traditions* https://twinlakesrecoverycenter.com/creating-new-sober-holiday-traditions/

- *Resiliency In Families Affected By Addiction* https://www.addictionresource.net/substance-abuse-in-families/resiliency/

www.ingramcontent.com/pod-product-compliance
Lightning Source LLC
Chambersburg PA
CBHW050808250726
48653CB00006B/2138